School Based & Pediatric Occupational Therapy Resource Series:

Motor & Sensory Exploration through Basic Arts & Crafts

Volume 9

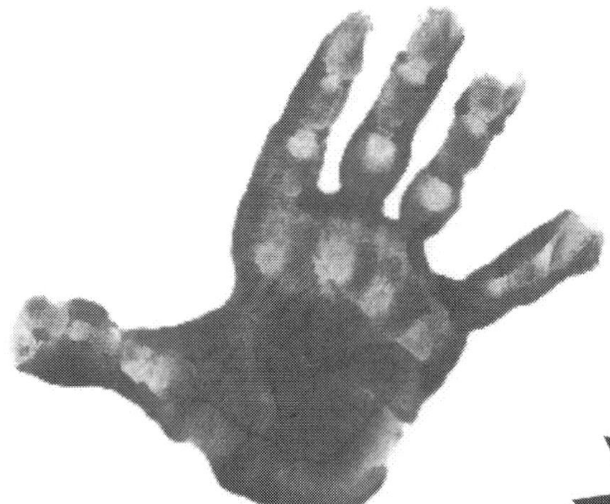

New! Updated Version with Sensory Integration and OT Practice Domain Framework.

By: S. Kelley, OTD, OTR/L

Purple Toes Books

Motor & Sensory Exploration through Basic Arts & Crafts
School Based & Pediatric Occupational Therapy Resource Series

by
S. Kelley, OTD, OTR/L

Purple Toes Books 2013

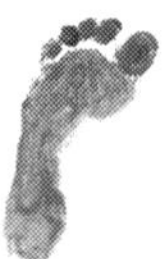

Dedication

This book is gratefully and gracefully dedicated to all the families and team members that I have shared in my journey.

This is for you.

Acknowledgements

This book and my work as an occupational therapist are made possible by the support and love of many wonderful people. I would like to thank my mentors, colleagues, and team members over the years, over the miles. Each experience has been unique and rewarding and I am thankful to have shared them with you.

I would like to acknowledge my husband for his unwavering support and love. To my parents and grandparents, you have provided me with the foundation for which I have remained grounded.

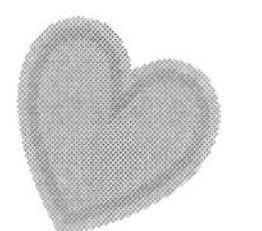

Special Thanks

To my son. Without your life, love and perseverance I would never know my own strength.

Let Go. Let God.

About the Author

Dr. S. Kelley, OTD, OTR/L currently practices as a pediatric occupational therapist in the school setting. She has facilitated the participation and skill growth for students in both regular education and special education programs. With a background as both an early childhood teacher and occupational therapist, Dr. Kelley has a unique and specialized perspective of education for students. Dr. Kelley specializes in the treatment of students in the early childhood self contained special education classes. After nearly 15 years of practice, Dr. Kelley decided to create resources for the school based and pediatric therapist to help facilitate effective and efficient practice. These resources reflect both the OT Practice Framework (AOTA, 2008) and the Common Core Curriculum (Common Core Standards Initiative, 2012). These resources were then made available in alternative formats for families and parents as a response from families and co-workers.

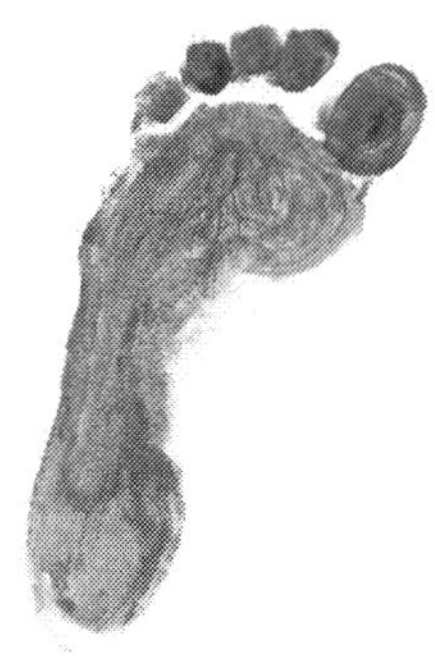

About Purple Toes Books

The purpose of my books, in various formats, is to provide the reader a collection of practice, easy-to-use activities to assist with various motor, language and social skills. This book, as well as all the others I've created, is a result of over 15 years of practice in pediatric occupational therapy. Over the course of my practice, I have created, developed, borrowed, collaborated, brainstormed, altered and modified countless activities and tasks. I decided to create a written series of my favorite activities as I use them, in the classroom, in the home or in the clinic.

Although I encourage you to read this book and independently apply the activities and/or interventions in your daily practice, classroom or life, please remind yourself that professionals are available to help you if you need advice or direction. These books are designed to be easy-to-use, but various professionals can help with modifications or adaptations if you need them.

Table of Contents

Occupational Therapy in School Setting

Definition of OT in the School Environment

Occupational therapists promote functional activities and engagement of daily routines. Areas of occupation including, but are not limited to: work, play, leisure, and social participation, ADL, IADLs and Education. According to IDEA, occupational therapy services in the school setting are a support services for students identified eligible for special education services. Under Part B of IDEA (2004), services are provided through the individual education plan (IEP) to promote academic success and social participation , to access, progress and participation in the educational environment in the least restrictive environment (AOTA, 2012). Under IDEA's Part B (2004) Regulation the Definition of Occupational Therapy includes the following components:

1. Services must be provided by a qualified occupational therapist
2. Services may "improve, develop or restore functions impaired or lost through illness, injury or deprivation"
3. Services may "improve the ability to perform tasks for independent functioning if functions are impaired or lost"
4. Services may "prevent, through early intervention, initial or further impairment or loss of function" (IDEA, 2004)

OT Goals & Outcomes

Through direct, collaborative and consultative services, occupational therapist create individualized goals with focus on outcomes related to:

1. General Classroom Skills/Accessibility/Participation
2. Playground and Sports Accessibility/Participation
3. School Based Self Help Skills
4. Social Participation in the School Setting
5. Mobility in the educational environment
6. Social Emotional Learning
7. Assistive technology in the educational setting
8. Sensory Regulation
9. Pre-vocational and Vocational Needs in the educational setting

Specific Services Occupational Therapists in the School Setting

- Evaluate students' strengths and weaknesses
- Identify modifications to promote participation
- Provide direct interventions to facilitate function and skill acquisition
- Collaborate and consult with teachers and staff regarding student needs to access his/her educational environment

All Student Support Systems

Occupational therapists in the school setting may provide support services for students with and without disability. This is done through early intervening services, including Response to Intervention.

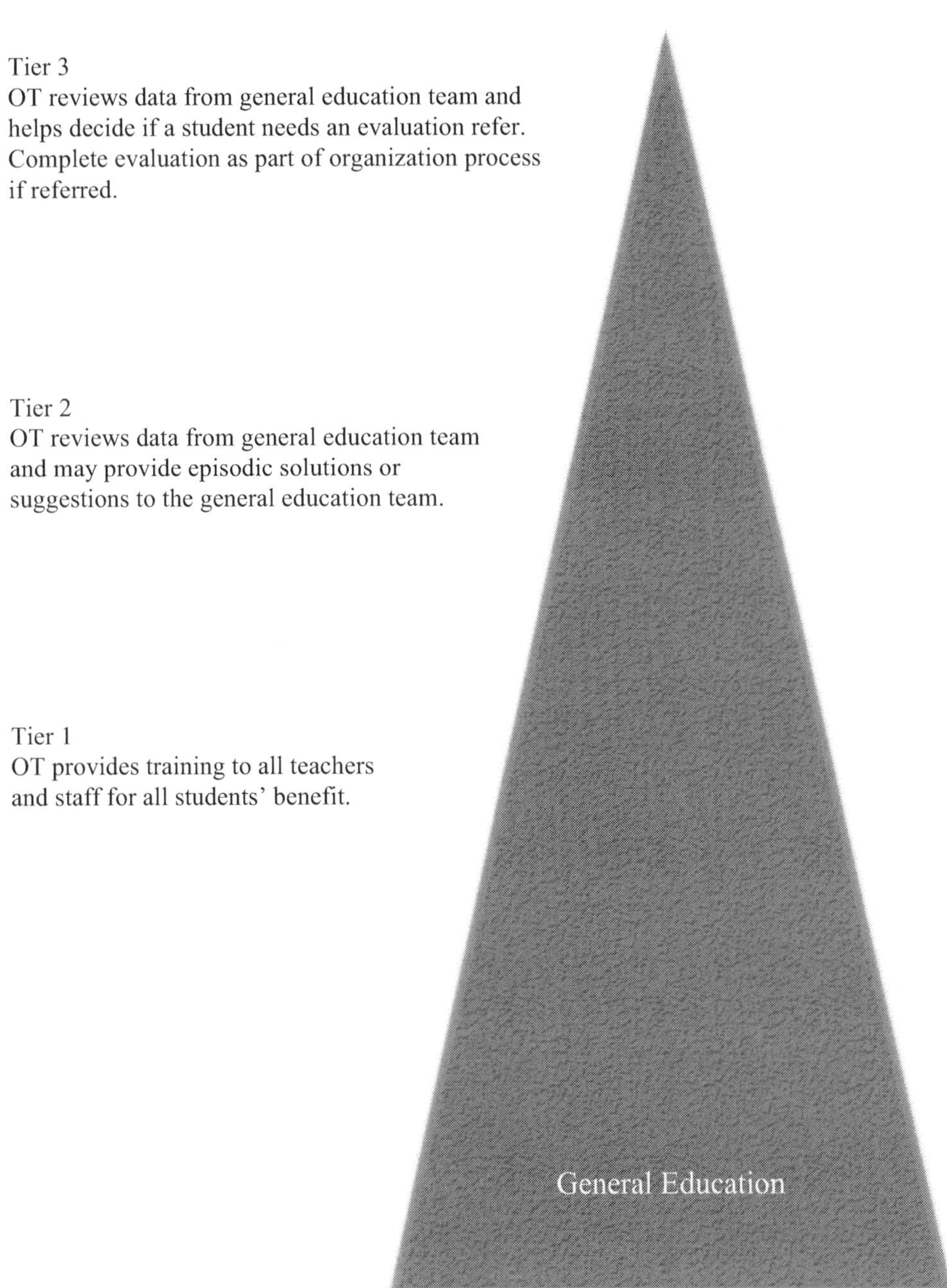

Application of the OT Practice Framework: Domain and Process

This book provides an individual and group method to provide services for students with and without disability. Below are the components reflected in the OT Practice Framework (AOTA, 2008) that are potential outcomes of the group treatment.

After the students' occupational profile has been developed, this group serves as the intervention plan, implementation and review within the intervention process. The intervention process includes the following (AOTA, 2008):

- Plan: Guides the actions of the OT and is based on the students' priorities
- Interventions: Carried out actions that address performance skills, patterns, context, activity demands and client factors that are impacting performance
- Review: Allow for revisions in the plan and actions

It should be noted, all interventions have the primary goal to achieving the primary outcome of engagement in occupation to support participation. (AOTA, 2008)

Areas of Occupation

Education
Play
Leisure
Social Participation

Performance Skills

Motor Skills
- Posture (Stabilizes, Aligns, Positions)
- Mobility (Walks, Reaches, Bends)
- Coordination (Coordinates, Manipulates, Flows)
- Strength & Effort (Moves, Transport, Lifts, Calibrates, Grips)
- Energy (Endures, Paces)

Process Skills
- Energy (Paces, Attends)
- Knowledge (Chooses, Uses, Handles, Heeds, Inquires)
- Temporal Organization (Initiates, Continues, Sequences, Terminates)
- Organizing Space & Objects (Searches, Gathers)

Intervention Plan for Groups

Occupational Therapy Intervention Approach

Create/Promote – performance skills, activity demands
Establish/Restore – performance skills
Maintain – performance skills, activity demands

Mechanism for Service Delivery

OT will provide the intervention with the support of additional team members which may include a speech language pathologist, physical therapist, teacher and/or support staff in the classroom

Each intervention or group should be delivered one time; however, the teacher or team may decide to expand the concept if additional practice is warranted. Additionally, group or intervention plans are designedto be delivered at least weekly. Groups should be implemented for about twenty to thirty minutes.

Outcome Measures & Types of Outcomes

Long term goal is to promote and facilitate the engagement in occupation. "Engagement in occupation (education or play) to support participation is the broad outcome of intervention that is designed to foster performance in desired and needed occupations or activities" (AOTA, 2008, p. 627).

Each group focus on the outcome of occupational performance (access to education).

Therapeutic Use of Self

The therapist uses his/her own personality, insight, perception and judgments throughout the intervention. Each group or activity requires the therapist to use his/herself to be a part of the intervention.

Therapeutic Use of Occupations and Activities

Each group or activity uses the following -
Occupational-Based Activity: Use of actual occupations as part of the intervention to support the outcome
Purposeful Activity: Use of goal-directed behaviors and activities in a therapeutically designed task

Application of the Sensory Integration Framework

Sensory Integration is defined as the organization of sensory input from one's environment and the responses one's body has as a result. It is a complex system that requires the nervous system to work in harmony together to interact with the environment and experiences within it.

Vestibular Response: Sensation from body regarding gravity and movement (knowing where one's head is in space)

Proprioception Response: Sensation from the body, muscles and joints (where the body "feels" itself in space

Tactile/Touch: Feeling through the body, hands, skin

Visual Sense: Seeing what's in space and distinguishing between various visual input

Auditory Sense: Hearing sounds in space and distinguishing between various sound input

Olfactory Sense: Smelling scents in space and distinguishing between various smells

Gustatory Sense: Tasting food in the mouth and distinguishing between different tastes (sour, sweet, etc)

Dysfunctional Response: Negative action or emotional response, lack of response or mismatched response

Adaptations and Modifications to Support Participation

Adaptation Defined

An adaptation is HOW the student accesses information in the classroom

Modification Defined

An modification is WHAT the student is expected to learn in the classroom.

Hierarchy of Accommodations & Modifications

Most special education students may need Level 2 & 3

Level	Accommodations	Modifications
1	All students complete same activities	No changes made to success criteria
2	All students complete same activities, additional support and reinforcement needed	No changes made to success criteria
3	All students complete basic concept, but significant changes made to how it is learned	Success criteria changed slightly
4	Students complete a smaller part of the expected activity	Success criteria based on individual needs
5	Students complete alternative activity	Success criteria based on individual needs

Adaptations for Activity Sessions

Environment

- Provide organized and predictable space.
- Provide and reinforce rules and expectations.
- Create visual cues for rules and expectations.
- Create visuals for objects in the classroom.
- Remove visual clutter from space.
- Provide consistent expectations.
- Place students in a learning space that is removed from major distractions (doorway, pencil sharpener, distracting peers)
- Use visual behavior cue cards to redirect behaviors (stop, listen, look, quiet mouth)
- Distribute and encourage sensory tools for sensory seeking behaviors while seated
- Allow the use of noise cancelling headphones or earplugs for disruptions

Instruction

- Introduce basic concepts immediately before starting activity
- Reinforce concepts with frequent direction, redirection and questions
- Use manipulatives and movements
- Rephrase and repeat key concepts
- Reinforce vocabulary and concepts frequently
- Infuse discussion and instruction with desired concepts and vocabulary
- Reduce tasks to main concepts and components
- Focus on main concepts – eliminate extra information
- Move to a closer proximity to students when instructing

Fine Motor Specific

Experiment with:

Various grippers to improve control or grasping pattern
Weighted pencils for shaky marks (decreased motor control)
Vary the length or thickness of utensil
Vary type of utensil
Texture under paper (sandpaper)
Vary line sizes – start wider and get smaller
Raised line paper to cue base and top lines
Created raised line paper with glue
Skip every other line on paper
Enlarging paper to make fill in blanks larger
Experiment with adapted scissors – loop, mounted
Highlight desired fill in area
Provide stickers for a quick way to label work (instead of writing it)
Reduce written work required
Allow additional time to write
Provide near point from which to copy versus far point
Chair with side supports
Slant board
Label marker for spelling requirements
Recorder for oral responses vs written requirements
Word processor
Computer with voice recognition

Specific Motor, Sensory, & Language Skills Addressed

Motor Skills

Bi-Lateral Integration – Use of two hands together
In Hand Manipulation Skills
Finger Isolation
Grasping Patterns
Midline Crossing
Trunk Elongation, Strength and Stability
Postural Control
Wrist Rotation, Strength and Control
Hand Dominance
Breath Support
Jaw Stabilization
Lip Closure
Tongue Elevation and Movements

Sensory Skills

Vestibular Input
Proprioceptive
Tactile
Visual
Auditory
Gustatory

Language Skills

Sound Recognition
Greeting Peers
Requesting Materials
Turn Taking

Introduction

This book is intended to provide therapists, teachers and parents fun, easy crafts to explore to expand fine motor and sensory skills. The crafts are separated into three sections: scribble, painting and cut/paste. Some of the crafts are classics and some are fun new experiences to enjoy!

The time to complete tasks depends on the activity. Some take a few minutes and some can take longer. ENJOY!

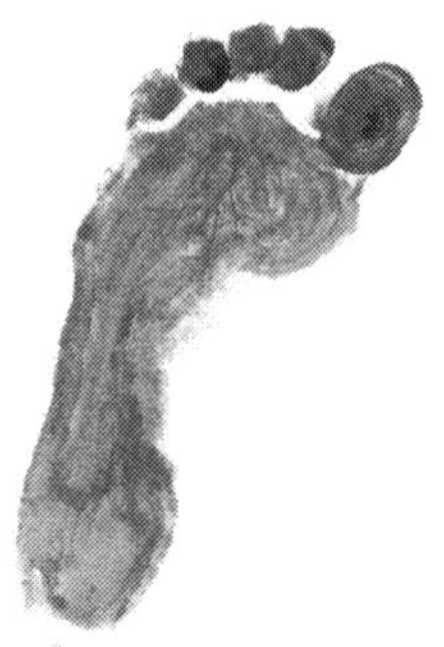

Materials

Chalk Play

Materials:
Colored chalk
Paper
Hair Spray

Melted Crayons

Materials:
Broken crayons (remove paper)
Muffin Pan
Oven
Aluminum Foil
White paper

Vertical Art

Materials:
Large white paper (butcher paper)
Tape
Crayons

Shadow Picture

Materials:
Desk lamp/flashlight
Table
White Paper
Markers, Crayons

Foot Prints

Materials:
Drawing paper
Crayon, colored pencils, markers
Glitter Glue

Thumbprints & Petals

Materials:
Washable stamp pad
White paper
Crayons/Markers

Connect the Stars

Materials:
Stars stickers
White Paper
Market/Crayons

Crayon Peek A Boo

Materials:
Various Crayons
Pencil
Sharp Pencil

Coffee Filter Color

Materials:
Washable markers
Coffer filter
Eyedropper

Fingerpaint Fingerprints

Materials:
Fingerpaint
White paper

Blue Boy Pictures

Materials:
Various shades of blue (4-5 different shades)
White Paper
Paintbrushes

Bingo Dot Painting

Materials:
Bingo Dabber/Do A Dots
Paper
Tape

Corn Shuck Painting

Materials:
Paint
Paper
Tape
Unshucked corn

Tissue Paper Painting

Materials:
Construction paper
Colored tissue paper squares
Scissors
Paintbrushes
Container of water

Salt Painting

Materials:
Dark colored construction paper
Crayons
Epson salts
Warm water (not too hot)
Measuring cups, bowls, spoon
Paintbrush

String Block Painting

Materials:
String/yarn
Small blocks of wood
Tempera Paint
Shallow Pan
Paper

Sponge Painting

Materials:
Scissors
Small thick sponges (cut into shapes)
Clothespins
Shallow paint pan
Paper

Fingerpainting

Materials:
Fingerpaint
Plastic Tabletop
Large sheets of paper

Roller Painting

Materials:
Thin Foam – Cut various shapes
Scissors
Glue
Empty paper towel or toilet paper roll (cardboard tube)
Tempera paint
Shallow Pan
Paper

Gadget Painting

Materials:
Empty Matchboxes
Small items (toothpicks, string, wood chips, curtain rings, bottle caps, cardboard shapes)
Glue
Paint
Shallow Paint Pan
Paper

Circle Circle Animals

Materials:
Various circles traced circles on colored paper
Scissors
Glue
Black marker/crayon

Me Puzzle

Materials:
Child (no smaller than 5X7)
Heavy paper
Glue
Scissors
Laminator

Paper Beads

Materials:
Scissors
Colored paper/tissue paper/gift wrap
Plastic straw
Glue
String

String Art

Materials:
Tempera paint
Liquid starch or glue
Small container
Scissors
String
Colored paper
White paper

Rice Picture

Materials:
Cotton Swab/Paintbrush
Glue
Heavy Paper
Rice

Funny Faces

Materials:
Old magazines
Scissors
Paper
Glue

Sugar Cube Buildings

Materials:
Sugar Cubes
Glue
Stryofoam meat trays
Paint

Playdough Jewelry

Materials:
Playdough
Toothpick
Clear nail polish
String

Spoon Art

Materials:
Wooden Kitchen Spoon
Glue
Yarn
Buttons
Markers

Paper Binoculars

Materials:
Two toilet paper rolls
Tape
Markers/Crayons/Stickers

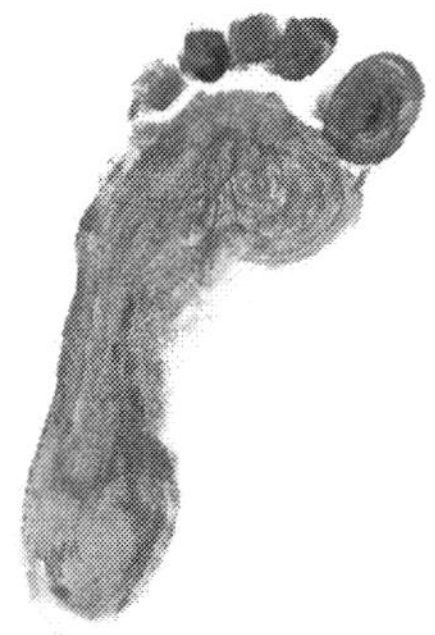

Arts and Crafts Plans

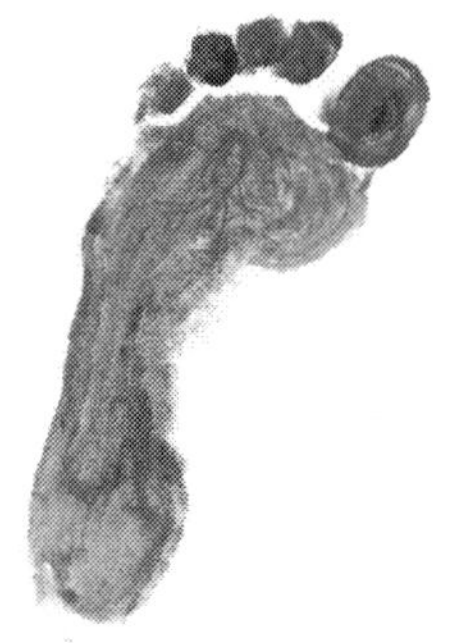

Scribble & Draw

Chalk Play

Materials:
Colored chalk
Paper
Hair Spray

Activity:

1. Use to chalk on white paper. Spray hair spray on chalk to “set it”.

2. Place white paper on textured surface. Use chalk to color over textures. Use hairspray to set chalk

Melted Crayons

Materials:
Broken crayons (remove paper)
Muffin Pan
Oven
Aluminum Foil
White paper

Activity:
Preheat oven to 400.
Line muffin pan with aluminum foil.
Put crayon pieces in muffin pan.
Place pan in oven and allow crayons to melt
Allow to cool completely
Pop out crayons and explore new crayons to draw on white paper

Vertical Art

Materials:
Large white paper (butcher paper)
Tape
Crayons

Activity:
Tape large paper to a vertical surface
Make sure it's stable enough for pressure from writing
Using crayons, draw and scribble on vertical surface
(Wall serves like an easel)

Shadow Picture

Materials:
Desk lamp/flashlight
Table
White Paper
Markers, Crayons

Activity:
Tape paper on the wall.
Position light so that a shadow can be cast on the paper.
Trace a shape with hands or trace facial silhouette

Foot Prints

Materials:
Drawing paper
Crayon, colored pencils, markers
Glitter Glue

Activity:
Stabilize white paper on flat surface.
Trace feet on white paper using crayons
Add glitter glue for "painted toes"

Thumbprints & Petals

Materials:
Washable stamp pad
White paper
Crayons/Markers

Activity:
Press thumb into stamp pad.
With ink on the thumb, then press the thumb onto the paper.
Demonstrate and encourage drawing petals around the thumb prints.

Connect the Stars

Materials:
Stars stickers
White Paper
Market/Crayons

Activity:
Position and stabilize white paper on vertical or horizontal surface
Peel and stick star stickers on paper in a random order
Connect the stars to create line art

Crayon Peek A Boo

Materials:
Various Crayons
Pencil
Sharp Pencil

Activity:
Color all over the white paper.
Color black all over the colored area
Use pencil to “carve” black crayon marking to reveal colors underneath

Coffee Filter Color

Materials:
Washable markers
Coffer filter
Eyedropper

Activity:
Place protective paper or plastic plate
Color with marker on coffee filter
Squeeze water on the coffee filter using eyedropper

Fingerpaint Fingerprints

Materials:
Fingerpaint
White paper

Activity:
Protect the work surface
Stabilize white paper
Choose paint color and help drop paint on paper.
Smear and create art with fingerpaint.

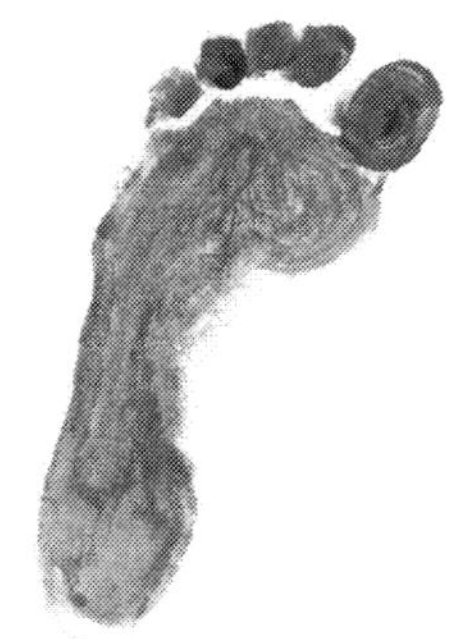

Paint

Blue Boy Pictures

Materials:

Various shades of blue (4-5 different shades)
White Paper
Paintbrushes

Activity:

Review the poem “Little Boy Blue”
Protect work area
Stabilize white paper on work area.
Paint with the various shades of blue.

Bingo Dot Painting

Materials:
Bingo Dabber/Do A Dots
Paper
Tape

Activity:
Prepare work area to protect furniture
Stabilize white paper in work area
Use dot paint to "dot dot dot" paper (muscle gradation is required to prevent too much paint from coming out)

Corn Shuck Painting

Materials:

Paint
Paper
Tape
Unshucked corn

Activity:

Prepare work area.
Help child shuck corn.
Use corn shuck to dip into paint and use the shucks to paint on paper.
Use corn cobs to roll into paint and paint on paper

Tissue Paper Painting

Materials:
Construction paper
Colored tissue paper squares
Scissors
Paintbrushes
Container of water

Activity:
Lay out pieces of construction paper on protected area.
Secure paper.
Use paint brushes to “paint” water all over construction paper.
Put tissue paper squares on top of watered construction paper.
Paint tissue paper with water again.
Remove tissue paper.

Salt Painting

Materials:

Dark colored construction paper
Crayons
Epson salts
Warm water (not too hot)
Measuring cups, bowls, spoon
Paintbrush

Activity:

Boil 2 cups of water and put 1 cup of Epson salt into boiling water to dissolve.
Color pictures with crayons on dark colored paper.
Press hard with crayons (apply heavy pressure)
Cool Epson salt water and use paintbrush to paint over picture.
Cover the picture several times with Epson salt solution
Dry.

String Block Painting

Materials:
String/yarn
Small blocks of wood
Tempera Paint
Shallow Pan
Paper

Activity:
Wrap string around wooden block.
Tie in place.
Press string block into a pan of paint.
Press string block onto paper to create a design

Sponge Painting

Materials:
Scissors
Small thick sponges (cut into shapes)
Clothespins
Shallow paint pan
Paper

Activity:
Clip clothespins on the top of sponges
Press sponges into shallow paint pan using the clothespin "handle"
Transfer sponge from pan to white paper to make picture

Fingerpainting

Materials:
Fingerpaint
Plastic Tabletop
Large sheets of paper

Activity:
Protect work area.
Secure paper to work area.
Explore finger paints by moving paint around with fingers all over white paper.

Roller Painting

Materials:
Thin Foam – Cut various shapes
Scissors
Glue
Empty paper towel or toilet paper roll (cardboard tube)
Tempera paint
Shallow Pan
Paper

Activity:
Protect work area.
Secure white paper in work area.
Glue foam shapes on cardboard tube
Pour small amount of paint into pan
Dip roller into pan
Roll onto a sheet of paper

Gadget Painting

Materials:
Empty Matchboxes
Small items (toothpicks, string, wood chips, curtain rings, bottle caps, cardboard shapes)
Glue
Paint
Shallow Paint Pan
Paper

Activity:
Glue shapes onto empty matchboxes
Press matchboxes into shallow paint pan
Transfer matchbox from paint pan to paper to create picture

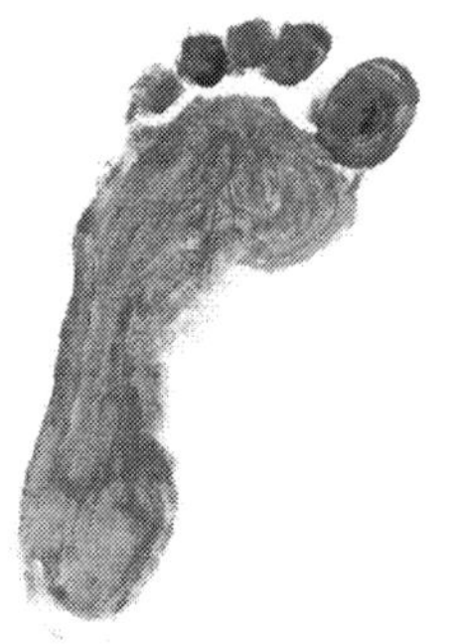

Glue, Paper & Scissors

Circle Circle Animals

Materials:

Various circles traced circles on colored paper
Scissors
Glue
Black marker/crayon

Activity:

Practice cutting out all the various circles
Cut some circles in half
Glue circles and semi-circles in animal shapes

* Adapt this task by changing shape: triangle or square

Me Puzzle

Materials:

Child (no smaller than 5X7)
Heavy paper
Glue
Scissors
Laminator

Activity:

Glue photo to heavy paper and laminate.
Help child cut photo into several pieces (number of pieces depends on child's ability/age)
Practice putting the photo

Paper Beads

Materials:
Scissors
Colored paper/tissue paper/gift wrap
Plastic straw
Glue
String

Activity:
Cut paper the size of the drinking straw and about 2 inches wide.
Spread glue all over straw and then apply paper (roll it one)
Let the glue dry and cut straw into ½ inch pieces
The paper beads are created and string can be threaded through to create a neckalce

String Art

Materials:

Tempera paint
Liquid starch or glue
Small container
Scissors
String
Colored paper
White paper

Activity:

Mix equal parts paint and glue and put into container.
Cut string into various length
Dip strings into paint container
Arrange paint string on colored paper to make a design

Rice Picture

Materials:
Cotton Swab/Paintbrush
Glue
Heavy Paper
Rice

Activity:
Dip the paintbrush into the glue and brush it on paper.
Sprinkle rice on the glue.
Shake paper to remove the excess rice

Funny Faces

Materials:
Old magazines
Scissors
Paper
Glue

Activity:
Find various photos of faces and cut out eyes, nose, mouths, ears and heads and cut
Glue mixed up face parts on white paper.

Sugar Cube Buildings

Materials:

Sugar Cubes
Glue
Stryofoam meat trays
Paint

Activity:

Glue sugar cube squares on a stryofoam base.
Be creative!

Playdough Jewelry

Materials:
Playdough
Toothpick
Clear nail polish
String

Activity:
Roll playdough into small balls and puncture ball with toothpick (large enough hole for string)
Allow playdough to dry for several days
Once dry, paint with clear nail polish
Allow to dry.
Thread bead on string

Spoon Art

Materials:

Wooden Kitchen Spoon
Glue
Yarn
Buttons
Markers

Activity:

Create spoon person by:
Yarn for hair
Buttons for eyes
Markers create nose and mouth
More spoons can be used for more family members

Paper Binoculars

Materials:

Two toilet paper rolls
Tape
Markers/Crayons/Stickers

Activity:

Tape two rolls together like binoculars
Decorate the binoculars with markers, crayons or stickers

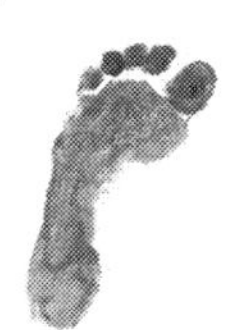

Additional Resources from Purple Toes Books

Written by an OT for OTs, teachers and families!

For Occupational Therapists

Quick Fine Motor and Sensory Screener and Assessment
Groups to Facilitate Motor and Language Skills with Classroom Materials
Groups to Facilitate Motor, Sensory and Language Skills 2
Group Sensory Experiences
Sensory Experiences Through Play
Early Intervention Play
Fine Motor Items for Play
MORE! Early Intervention Play for Infants and Toddlers
MORE! Fine Motor Items for Play

For Teachers

Groups to Facilitate Motor and Language Skills with Classroom Materials
Groups to Facilitate Motor, Sensory and Language Skills 2
Classroom Group Sensory Experiences
Sensory Experiences Through Play in the Classroom
Early Intervention Play for the Developmental Therapist and Teacher
Fine Motor Items for Daily Practice
MORE! Early Intervention Play for Infants and Toddlers
MORE! Fine Motor Items for Daily Practice

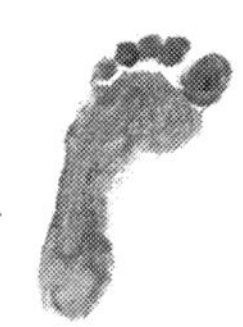

Additional Resources from Purple Toes Books

Written by an OT for OTs, teachers and families!

For Parents

Activities to Facilitate Motor and Language Skills with Household Materials
Activities to Facilitate Motor, Sensory and Language Skills 2
Play Date Sensory Experiences
More! Play Date Sensory Experiences
Early Intervention Play Time
Fine Motor Daily Practice
MORE! Early Intervention Play Time with Infants and Toddlers
MORE! Fine Motor Daily Practice

More books slated for publication….

Check out PurpleToesBooks.com or Amazon for details!

School Based & Pediatric Occupational Therapy Resource Series Book Listing

These are clinical resource books for school based or clinic based occupational therapists. The materials created are actual materials used by Dr. Kelley in her practice and have been integrated as part of her practice for over fifteen years. Dr. Kelley has divided her focus for each book into areas of focus for the therapists. Reflecting the Occupational Therapy Practice Domain (AOTA, 2008), the activities seek to address components as they are outlined in the Domain. As a collaboration of many resources, experiences and personal development, the OT Resources Series is designed by an OT for an OT.

Volume 1: ***Groups to Facilitate Motor and Language Skills with Classroom Materials***
Groups for early childhood and elementary students or clinic-based treatments (can be adjusted for any age/ability group) to facilitate fine motor, gross motor, language and social skills

Volume 2: ***Groups to Facilitate Motor, Sensory and Language Skills 2***
MORE! Groups for early childhood and elementary (can be adjusted for any age/ability group) to facilitate fine motor, gross motor, language and social skills
Integrates the use of a puppet
Provides specific greeting protocol for group start and end to promote eye contact and engagement

Volume 3: ***Group Sensory Experiences***
Fun, basic sensory groups for various age groups
Primary focus on motor planning (praxis), proprioception and vestibular input, with integration of other sensory systems

Volume 4: ***Sensory Experiences Through Play***
Play activities for various age groups
Focus on all sensory systems through exploratory play, structured guided play and imaginary play

Volume 5: ***Early Intervention Play***

Designed for early intervention aged students or clients, these activities are designed to facilitate sensory experiences at a basic and introductory level. These tasks can be adapted for various age groups if needs depending on skill level

Volume 6: *Fine Motor Items for Play*
Basic, pictured fine motor tasks designed for daily use for your child and/or student. Each task is aligned with fine motor and sensory performance skills and can be adapted for various age and ability levels. A calendar for reference is provided to incorporate into intervention plans.

Volume 7: *MORE! Early Intervention Play for Infants & Toddlers*
Designed for early intervention aged students or clients, these activities are designed to facilitate basic play experiences at a basic and introductory level. These tasks can be adapted for various age groups if needs depending on skill level, but are very basic in nature for the infant and toddler's developmental level.

Volume 8: *MORE! Fine Motor Items for Play*
Basic, easy fine motor items designed for daily fine motor play for your child and/or student. Each task can be aligned with fine motor and sensory performance skills and can be adapted for various age and ability levels

Volume 9: *Motor & Sensory Exploration through Basic Arts & Crafts*
The purpose of *Motor & Sensory Exploration through Basic Arts & Crafts* is to provide therapists, teachers or families easy, quick crafts to incorporate into groups or treatment for fine motor and sensory practice and development. This book includes three sections: Scribbling, Paint & Cut/Paste.

Volume 10: *MORE! Motor & Sensory Exploration through Basic Arts & Crafts*
The purpose of *MORE! Motor & Sensory Exploration through Basic Arts & Crafts* is to provide therapists, teachers or families easy, quick crafts to incorporate into groups or treatment for fine motor and sensory practice and development. This book includes three sections: Scribbling, and Edible Crafts.

Volume 11: *HOLIDAY & SEASONS! Motor & Sensory Exploration through Basic Arts & Crafts*

Third of the Craft Series, *HOLIDAY & SEASON! Motor & Sensory Exploration through Basic Arts & Crafts* provides therapists, teachers or families easy, quick crafts to incorporate into groups or treatment for fine motor and sensory practice and development.

Volume 12: *Therapeutic Cooking Groups for Early Learners*
Cooking Groups are an excellent way to incorporate various fine motor, language and sensory experiences into one task. This book provides 34 thematically based cooking tasks. Each task is broken up into no more than six steps per task making visual cueing easy to create. The cooking tasks included in this book are actual tasks used in the classroom and therapy setting.

Volume 13: *MORE! Therapeutic Cooking Groups for Early Learners*
Cooking Groups are an excellent way to incorporate various fine motor, language and sensory experiences into one task. This book provides 34 MORE thematically based cooking tasks. Each task is broken up into no more than six steps per task making visual cueing easy to create. The cooking tasks included in this book are actual tasks used in the classroom and therapy setting

Volume 14: *Therapeutic Play with Classroom & Home Items*
Using basic household items, this book, *Therapeutic Play with Classroom & Home Items,* provides various tasks and activities for individual and group play. Items for play included are: newspaper, cardboard boxes, paper, lids and tops, small containers, yarn/string and cans. Six specific skills are addressed for each item.

Special Edition: *Quick Pediatric Fine Motor and Sensory Screener and Assessment*
Practical Fine Motor Screener and Data Collection
Includes a Basic Sensory Screener

Also check out the Teacher and Parent versions of these books!

Http://www.purpletoesbooks.com

References

American Occupational Therapy Association. (2008). Occupational therapy practice framework: Domain and process (2nd ed.). American Journal of Occupational Therapy , 62, 625–683.

American Occupational Therapy Association (2012). Role of Occupational Therapy with Children and Youth with Children and Youth in School in School-Based Practice.

Ayres, A. J. (2005). *Sensory integration and the child: 25th anniversary edition.* Lost Angeles, CA: Western Psychological Services.

Individuals With Disabilities Education Act, 20 U.S.C. § 1400 (2004).

Made in the USA
Columbia, SC
01 April 2024